The Wellness Lifestyle Workbook

Self-Assessments, Exercises & Educational Handouts

Ester A. Leutenberg
John J. Liptak, EdD

Illustrated by
Amy L. Brodsky, LISW

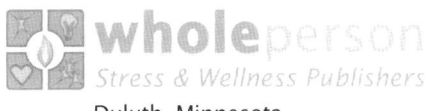

Duluth, Minnesota

Whole Person
101 W. 2nd St., Suite 203
Duluth, MN 55802

800-247-6789

books@wholeperson.com
www.wholeperson.com

The Wellness Lifestyle Workbook
Self-Assessments, Exercises & Educational Handouts

Copyright ©2009 by Ester A. Leutenberg and John J. Liptak.
All rights reserved. Except for short excerpts for review purposes and materials in the assessment, journaling activities, and educational handouts sections, no part of this book may be reproduced or transmitted in any form by any means, electronic or mechanical, including photocopying without permission in writing from the publisher.

Printed in the United States of America

10 9 8 7 6 5 4 3 2 1

Editorial Director: Carlene Sippola
Art Director: Joy Morgan Dey

Library of Congress Control Number: 2009925430
ISBN: 978-1-57025-233-4

Using This Book *(For the professional)*

Wellness and health are interrelated, but distinct concepts. Health is considered freedom from disease; it is the condition in which people are able to do their most constructive work, provide the best possible service to the world, and experience the highest possible enjoyment in leisure-time experiences. *Wellness*, on the other hand, is much more complex than basic physical health. *Wellness* is the ability to fully integrate physical, mental, emotional, social, and spiritual well-being into an effective lifestyle. Optimum wellness balances the following five basic dimensions:

Physical Dimension – This dimension is related to sound nutritional practices, maintaining proper weight, participating in regular exercise, getting enough sleep, engaging in physical activity, avoiding risky behavior, and restricting intake of harmful substances.

Career Dimension – This dimension is related to finding balance among various life roles as people engage in fulfilling work and related activities, and identifying leisure activities that will provide a sense of life satisfaction.

Emotional Dimension – This dimension is related to understanding personal feelings, maintaining a relatively even emotional state, accepting one's own limitations, expressing emotions effectively, adjusting to change, and maintaining good, healthy relationships with other people.

Social Dimension – This dimension is related to sharing friendships, family relationships and group memberships. It entails using empathy and active listening skills, caring genuinely about other people, being open to caring from other people, and committing to the common good of the community, nation, and world.

Spiritual Dimension – This dimension is related to maintaining a sense that life is meaningful, employing a continuing quest for value and purpose, searching for clarity, committing to peace and contentment in life, and developing the fortitude to continue in the face of obstacles.

A wellness lifestyle pervades all aspects of a person's life independent and with others in school, work, leisure, community activities and in a group. A wellness lifestyle helps to minimize stress and promote well-being and self-fulfillment. The notion of wellness suggests that people are whole beings, not fragmented parts that can be dealt with separately. Wellness stresses conscious effort and commitment to one's ability to resist disease and maintain optimum health.

(Continued)

Using This Book (For the professional, continued)

The Wellness Lifestyle Workbook contains five separate sections and a bonus section to help participants learn more about themselves and their lifestyles. They will learn about a wellness lifestyle that promotes health and well-being.

The sections of this book are:

1) **COPING WITH STRESS SCALE** helps individuals identify their basic style for dealing with stress.

2) **PHYSICAL FITNESS SCALE** helps individuals identify if they are eating well, getting plenty of relaxation sleep and exercising regularly in order to be able to cope effectively with stress.

3) **CREATIVE LEISURE SCALE** helps individuals explore their leisure interests and creative ways of implementing these interests in productive activities.

4) **HEALTHY RELATIONSHIPS SCALE** helps individuals determine whether they have developed a healthy intimate relationship with their partners and productive relationships with family members.

5) **SPIRITUAL WELLNESS SCALE** helps individuals explore how spiritually well they currently are.

BONUS — LIFE SKILLS SCALE helps individuals identify major strengths and weaknesses in the life skills they possess.

These sections serve as avenues for individual self-reflection, as well as for group experiences revolving around identified topics of importance. Each assessment includes directions for easy administration, scoring and interpretation. Each section includes exploratory activities, reflective journaling activities and educational handouts to help participants discover their habitual effective and ineffective methods of managing health and wellness and exploring new ways to bring about healing.

The art of self-reflection goes back many centuries and is rooted in many of the world's greatest spiritual and philosophical traditions. Socrates, the ancient Greek philosopher, was known to walk the streets engaging the people he met in philosophical reflection and dialogue. He felt that this type of activity was so important in life that he went so far as to proclaim, "The unexamined life is not worth living!" The unexamined life is one in which the same routine is continually repeated without ever thinking about its meaning to one's life and how this life really could be lived. However, a structured reflection and examination of beliefs, assumptions, characteristics, and patterns can provide a better understanding, which can lead to a more satisfying life. A greater level of self-understanding about important life skills is often necessary to make positive, self-directed changes in the negative patterns that keep repeating. The assessments and exercises in this book can help promote this

Using This Book *(For the professional, continued)*

self-understanding. Through involvement in the in-depth activities, the participant claims ownership in the development of positive patterns.

Journaling is an extremely powerful tool for enhancing self-discovery, learning, transcending traditional problems, breaking ineffective life habits, and helping to heal from psychological traumas of the past. From a physical point of view, writing reduces stress and lowers muscle tension, blood pressure and heart rate levels. Psychologically, writing reduces sadness, depression and general anxiety, and leads to a greater level of life satisfaction and optimism. Behaviorally, writing leads to enhanced social skills, emotional intelligence and creativity. It also leads to improved writing skills which leads to more self-confidence in the workplace.

By combining reflective assessment and journaling, participants will be exposed to a powerful method of combining verbalizing and writing to reflect on and solve problems. Participants will become more aware of health and wellness issues in their lives.

Preparation for using the assessments and activities in this book is important. The authors suggest that prior to administering any of the assessments in this book, you complete them yourself. This will familiarize you with the format of the assessments, the scoring directions, the interpretation guides and the journaling activities. Although the assessments are designed to be self-administered, scored and interpreted. This familiarity will help prepare facilitators to answer questions about the assessments for participants.

The Assessments, Journaling Activities and Educational Handouts

The Assessments, Journaling Activities, and Educational Handouts in *The Wellness Lifestyle Workbook* are reproducible and ready to be photocopied for participants' use. Assessments contained in this book focus on self-reported data and are similar to ones used by psychologists, counselors, therapists and career consultants. Accuracy and usefulness of the information provided is dependent on the truthful information that each participant provides through self-examination. By being honest, participants help themselves to learn about unproductive and ineffective patterns, and to uncover information that might be keeping them from being as happy and/or as successful as they might be.

An assessment instrument can provide participants with valuable information about themselves; however, it cannot measure or identify everything about them. The purposes of the assessments are not to pigeon-hole certain characteristics, but rather to allow participants to explore all of their characteristics. This book contains self-assessments, not tests. Tests measure knowledge or whether something is right or wrong. For the assessments in this book, there are no right or wrong answers. These assessments ask for personal opinions or attitudes about a topic of importance in the participant's career and life.

When administering assessments in this workbook, remember that the items are generically written so that they will be applicable to a wide variety of people but will not account for every possible variable for every person. The assessments are not specifically tailored to one person. Use them to help participants identify possible negative themes in their lives and find ways to break the hold that these patterns and their effects have.

Advise the participants taking the assessments that they should not spend too much time trying to analyze the content of the questions; their initial response will most likely be true. Regardless of individual scores, encourage participants to talk about their findings and their feelings pertaining to what they have discovered about themselves. Talking about health, wellness, and overall well-being can enhance the life of participants. These wellness exercises can be used by group facilitators working with any populations who want to strengthen their overall wellness.

A particular score on any assessment does not guarantee a participant's level of health or wellness. Use discretion when using any of the information or feedback provided in this workbook. The use of these assessments should not be substituted for consultation and/or wellness planning with a health care professional.

Thanks to the following professionals whose input in this book has been so valuable!

Kathy Khalsa, OTR/L
Kathy Liptak, Ed.D.

Eileen Regen, M.Ed., CJE
Lucy Ritzic, OTR/L

Layout of the Book

This book includes:

- **Assessment Instruments** – Self-assessment inventories with scoring directions and interpretation materials. Group facilitators can choose one or more of the activities relevant to their participants.
- **Activity Handouts** – Practical questions and activities that prompt self-reflection and promote self-understanding. These questions and activities foster introspection and promote pro-social behaviors.
- **Reflective Questions for Journaling** – Self-exploration activities and journaling exercises specific to each assessment to enhance self-discovery, learning and healing.
- **Educational Handouts** – Handouts designed to enhance instruction can be used individually or in groups. They can be distributed, converted into masters for overheads or transparencies, or written down on a board and discussed.

Who should use this program?

This book has been designed as a practical tool for helping professional therapists, counselors, psychologists, teachers, group leaders, etc. Depending on the role of the professional using *The Wellness Lifestyle Workbook* and the specific group's needs, these sections can be used individually, combined, or implemented as part of an integrated curriculum for a more comprehensive approach.

Why use self-assessments?

Self-assessments are important in teaching various health and wellness skills. Participants will:

- Become aware of the primary motivators that guide their behavior.
- Explore and learn to indentify potentially harmful situations.
- Explore the effects of messages received in childhood.
- Gain insight that will guide behavioral change.
- Focus thinking on behavioral goals for change.
- Uncover resources they possess that can help to cope with problems and difficulties.
- Explore personal characteristics without judgment.
- Develop full awareness of personal strengths and weaknesses.

Because the assessments are presented in a straightforward and easy-to-use format, individuals can self-administer, score, and interpret each assessment independently.

Introduction for the Participant

Wellness practitioners and researchers believe that your health lies on a continuum and is an ever-changing balance between your physical, mental, emotional, social, and spiritual dimensions. Jesse Williams, one of the pioneers of the health education movement, suggested that health as freedom from disease was not a sufficient description, and that health should be seen as a quality of life and a standard of inspiration and increasing achievements, as well as the energy to do the things one cares about. *

Wellness combines your physical, mental, emotional, social, and spiritual health into a quality way of life. Wellness is the ability to live your life to the fullest, have zest for life, experience joy in all you do, and maximize your full potential. As you can see, wellness includes much more than just your physical health.

Most people are not proactive in their approach to wellness; they simply wait for disease to strike them, then they consult a physician to treat the disease and the symptoms. People who subscribe to the notion of wellness, on the other hand, take responsibility for their health and are continually learning about themselves and making the changes that will enhance their state of wellness. Now is the time for you to take charge of your life and make changes (sometimes drastic changes) that will make you healthier, prevent disease, and enhance your overall wellness. This book, The Wellness Lifestyle Workbook, is designed to help you learn more about yourself, discover how to balance all of your health dimensions, and improve your overall feeling of wellness and well-being.

*Williams, J. F. (1964). The Administration of Health Education & Physical Education. *St. Louis, MO: W.B. Saunders / Elsevier.*

The Wellness Lifestyle Workbook
TABLE OF CONTENTS

Section I: Coping with Stress Scale

Coping with Stress Scale
    Coping with Stress Scale Directions 15
    Coping with Stress Scale 16
    Coping with Stress Scale Scoring Directions 18
    Coping with Stress Scale Profile Interpretation 19–22

Exercises
    Stressful Situations in Which I Have Successfully Coped ... 23–24
    Stress Management Worksheet 25–26

Journaling Activities
    Your Stress Management Style 27

Educational Handouts
    Ways of Coping with Stress 28
    Tips for Coping with Stress 29

Section II: Physical Fitness Scale

Physical Fitness Scale
    Physical Fitness Scale Directions 33
    Physical Fitness Scale 34–35
    Physical Fitness Scale Scoring Directions 36
    Physical Fitness Scale Profile Interpretation 36

Exercises
    Sleep 37
    Things That Steal My Sleep 38
    Exercise 39–40
    Leisure-Time Physical Activity 41
    Setting Goals for Your Health 42
    My Goals 43
    Nutrition 44

Journaling Activities
    My Physical Fitness 45
    My Physical Fitness Benefits 46

Educational Handouts
    Eating Patterns and Links between Stress and Nutrition 47
    When You are Starting an Exercise Program 48

TABLE OF CONTENTS (continued)

Section III: Creative Leisure Scale

Creative Leisure Scale
    Creative Leisure Scale Directions 51
    Creative Leisure Scale 52–54
    Creative Leisure Scale Scoring Directions. 55
    Creative Leisure Scale Profile Interpretation. 56
    Creative Leisure Scale Descriptions 56–58

Exercises
    The Importance of Leisure 59
    Developmental Leisure Exercise 60
    Leisure Exploration 61
    Overcoming Barriers to Leisure Participation 62–63

Journaling Activities
    Leisure Activities 64

Educational Handouts
    Characteristics of Leisure. 65

Section IV: Healthy Relationships Scale

Healthy Relationships Scale
    Healthy Relationships Scale Directions 69
    Healthy Relationships Scale 70–71
    Healthy Relationships Scale Scoring Directions 72
    Healthy Relationships Scale Profile Interpretation 72

Exercises
    Partner Exploration 73
    Appreciation 74
    Relationship Philosophy. 75
    Conflict 76
    Sending Emotional Messages. 77–78
    Family and/or Friend Issues. 79
    Finances. 80

Journaling Activities
    Techniques. 81
    New Techniques. 82

TABLE OF CONTENTS (continued)

Educational Handouts
    Qualities of a Healthy Relationship 83

Section V: Spiritual Wellness Scale

Spiritual Wellness Scale
    Spiritual Wellness Scale Directions 87
    Spiritual Wellness Scale 88–89
    Spiritual Wellness Scale Scoring Directions 90
    Spiritual Wellness Scale Profile Interpretation. 90
    Spiritual Wellness Scale Descriptions 91

Exercises
    Spiritual Meditation 92
    Spiritual Writing 92
    Life Purpose. 93–94
    Discovering Your Purpose 95
    Forgiveness 96
    Spend Time in Nature 97
    Express Your Creativity 97
    Engage in Spiritual Practice 97
    Perform Community Service 97

Journaling Activities
    Family Influences. 98
    Spiritual Practices. 99

Educational Handouts
    Qualities of Spirituality. 100

BONUS Section: Life Scales Scale

Life Scales Scale
    Life Scales Scale Directions 103
    Life Scales Scale. 104–105
    Life Scales Scale Scoring Directions 106
    Life Scales Scale Profile Interpretation 106
    Life Scales Scale Descriptions 107

TABLE OF CONTENTS (continued)

Exercises
 Work / Leisure Balance............................ 108–109
 Ideas for Work / Leisure / Relationship Balance........... 110
 Time Management................................ 111–112
 Conflict Resolution — Where & When My Conflicts Occur ... 113
 Conflict Resolution Patterns............................ 114
 Money Matters....................................... 115
 Family Monthly Budget Workshop 116

Journaling Activities
 I Learned about How I Balance Work and Leisure.......... 117
 I Learned about How I Manage My Time 118
 I Learned about How I Manage Conflicts 119
 I Learned about How I Manage My Money............... 120

Educational Handouts
 Positive Life Skills................................... 121

SECTION I:
Coping with Stress Scale

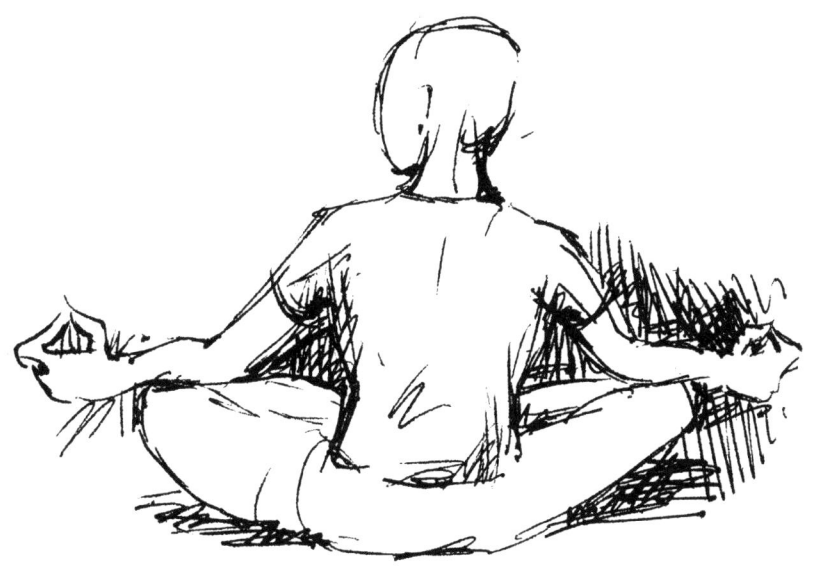

Name_____

Date_____

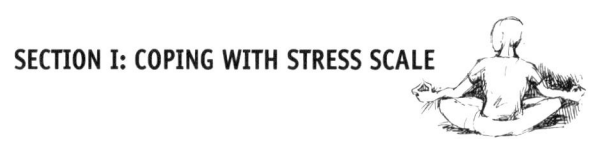

SECTION I: COPING WITH STRESS SCALE

Coping with Stress Scale Directions

Coping has been described as the efforts you use to manage specific internal and external stressors that tax your resources. Thus, coping is an ongoing process, and your repeated pattern of coping becomes your coping style.

People use many different strategies to cope with stress. All of the strategies have advantages and disadvantages. This assessment is designed to help you understand your approach to coping with stress in your life.

It contains 28 statements divided into four coping styles. Read each of the statements and decide whether or not the statement describes you. If the statement describes you, circle the **YES** next to the statement. If it does not describe you, circle the **NO** next to the statement.

In the following example, the circled **NO** indicates the statement is not descriptive of the person completing the inventory.

I take whatever actions I can to eliminate the stressor   YES   (NO)

This is not a test and there are no right or wrong answers. Do not spend too much time thinking about your answers. Your initial response will likely be the most true for you. Be sure to respond to every statement.

(Turn to the next page and begin)

SECTION I: COPING WITH STRESS SCALE

Coping with Stress Scale

When coping with a current stressor in my life . . .

SECTION I

I take whatever actions I can to eliminate the stressor	YES	NO
I do what has to be done, in a logical manner	YES	NO
I develop a strategy about what to do	YES	NO
I put aside other things and concentrate on the stressor	YES	NO
I don't allow myself to be distracted in dealing with the stressor	YES	NO
I seek to change the stressful situation	YES	NO
I change the physical stressor in the environment	YES	NO

TOTAL = _____

SECTION II

I work out	YES	NO
I use muscle relaxation techniques	YES	NO
I avoid using drugs, alcohol or stimulants to make myself feel better	YES	NO
I do deep breathing techniques	YES	NO
I continue to engage in healthy leisure activities	YES	NO
I organize my time effectively	YES	NO
I find entertainment to get my mind off the stressor	YES	NO

TOTAL = _____

(Continued on the next page)

SECTION I: COPING WITH STRESS SCALE

(Coping with Stress Scale, continued)

When coping with a current stressor in my life . . .

SECTION III

I find comfort in my spirituality	YES	NO
I get advice from people I trust	YES	NO
I talk to others to find out more about the situation	YES	NO
I use all of my available support systems	YES	NO
I communicate with trusted others about my feelings	YES	NO
I seek out people who have had similar experiences	YES	NO
I express my feelings in a socially acceptable manner	YES	NO

TOTAL = _____

SECTION IV

I attempt to focus on the positive side of the situation	YES	NO
I try to alter my irrational thinking	YES	NO
I try to turn the situation into an opportunity	YES	NO
I remind myself that the situation is temporary	YES	NO
I look for different ways to interpret the situation	YES	NO
I notice how my thinking is influencing the stress	YES	NO
I try to stop thinking about it so much	YES	NO

TOTAL = _____

(Go to the Scoring Directions on the next page)

SECTION I: COPING WITH STRESS SCALE

Coping with Stress Scale
Scoring Directions

This assessment is designed to measure your approach to coping with stress. Count the number of YES answers you circled in each section on the previous pages. Put that total on the line marked "Total" at the end of each section.

Then, transfer your totals to the spaces below:

SECTION I "TOTAL"   =   _____ (Behavioral)

SECTION II "TOTAL"   =   _____ (Physical)

SECTION III "TOTAL" =   _____ (Emotional)

SECTION IV "TOTAL"   =   _____ (Cognitive)

To be effective in coping with stress, you will probably use all four of the coping styles. The area or areas in which you scored the highest tend to be your most preferred coping style. Similarly, the area or areas in which you scored the lowest tend to be your least preferred coping style. Remember that the people who are most effective in coping with stress are able to effectively use all four styles well. Learning techniques from all four styles will help you deal with stressful situations. Notice your score for each of the sections and complete the activity handouts to better integrate techniques from each of the four styles in your life.

SECTION I: COPING WITH STRESS SCALE

Coping with Stress Scale
Profile Interpretation — Behavioral Coping Style

SCALE I — A BEHAVIORAL coping style is one in which you take action to eliminate the problems associated with the stressor in your environment. If you use this style you will develop an action strategy and concentrate on using the strategy to eliminate the stressor. You will seek out the stressor in your environment and make appropriate changes to eliminate the stressor.

List a time when this coping style has worked well for you.

_____
_____
_____
_____
_____

List a time when this coping style has not worked well for you.

_____
_____
_____
_____

Why did it work sometimes and other times did not? What was the difference?

_____
_____
_____
_____
_____

(Continued on the next page)

SECTION I: COPING WITH STRESS SCALE

Coping with Stress Scale
Profile Interpretation — Physical Coping Style

SCALE II — A PHYSICAL coping style is one in which you attempt to control the stress by engaging in physical activities and exercises. Some of the activities and exercises you may choose to engage in include working out in fitness center, using progressive relaxation techniques, avoiding stimulants, practicing deep breathing and continuing to engage in constructive leisure activities.

List a time when this coping style has worked well for you.

_____

_____

_____

_____

List a time when this coping style has not worked well for you.

_____

_____

_____

_____

Why did it work sometimes and other times did not? What was the difference?

_____

_____

_____

_____

(Continued on the next page)

Coping with Stress Scale
Profile Interpretation — Emotional Coping Style

SCALE III — AN EMOTIONAL coping style is one in which you reduce or eliminate stress by talking about your feelings. You find that talking to people in your support system, expressing your feelings, communicating with people who have been through the same type of thing, and seeking advice from people you trust, help you to reduce the stress in your life.

List a time when this coping style has worked well for you.

_____

_____

_____

_____

List a time when this coping style has not worked well for you.

_____

_____

_____

_____

Why did it work sometimes and other times did not? What was the difference?

_____

_____

_____

_____

(Continued on the next page)

SECTION I: COPING WITH STRESS SCALE

Coping with Stress Scale
Profile Interpretation — Cognitive Coping Style

SCALE IV — A COGNITIVE coping style is one in which you reduce the stress in your life by trying to control how you think about the situation. You try and keep a positive attitude, reduce the amount of irrational thinking you engage in, reframe how you see the stressful situation, look for various ways to interpret the stress, and search for opportunities in the stressful situation.

List a time when this coping style has worked well for you.

_____
_____
_____
_____

List a time when this coping style has not worked well for you.

_____
_____
_____
_____

Why did it work sometimes and other times did not? What was the difference?

_____
_____
_____
_____

SECTION I: ACTIVITY HANDOUTS

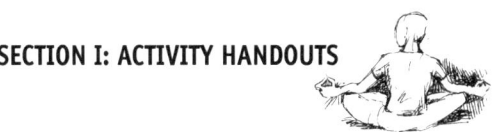

Becoming Skilled at Coping with Stress

You have successfully coped with stress and stressful situations in the past. These stressful situations may have been related to things happening with members of your family, in your relationships, your community, your job or school. List those stressful situations below and write down how you handled the stress using a variety of the techniques discussed in the assessment. Feel free to look back at the techniques listed in each of the four sections of the assessment. Then list what happened when you used these techniques.

Stressful Situations in Which I Have Successfully Coped

Example of when I used **BEHAVIORAL** techniques to cope with stress:

_____

_____

Outcome: _____

_____

Example of when I used **PHYSICAL** techniques to cope with stress:

_____

_____

Outcome: _____

_____

Example of when I used **EMOTIONAL** techniques to cope with stress:

_____

_____

Outcome: _____

_____

(Continued on the next page)

SECTION I: ACTIVITY HANDOUTS

Stressful Situations in Which I Have Successfully Coped (Continued)

Example of when I used **COGNITIVE** techniques to cope with stress:

_____

_____

Outcome: _____

_____

Review each of your examples, and identify the pros and cons of using each of the coping styles.

BEHAVIORAL _____

_____

_____

PHYSICAL _____

_____

_____

EMOTIONAL _____

_____

_____

COGNITIVE _____

_____

_____

SECTION I: ACTIVITY HANDOUTS

Stress Management Worksheet

Identify a stressful situation that you are currently encountering or you know is coming in the near future. Complete the following worksheet that will help you learn and apply the coping process:

1. Describe the situation.

_____

_____

2. Given the knowledge you have of yourself and the situation, describe why you find the situation stressful.

_____

_____

3. Decide how you can manage the situation in a way that it will not be so stressful.

_____

_____

4. What are the advantages and disadvantages of managing the stress — or letting the stress manage you?

_____

_____

5. What resources do you have for dealing with the situation?

_____

_____

(Continued on the next page)

SECTION I: ACTIVITY HANDOUTS

Stress Management Worksheet (Continued)

6. Take action using resources identified in the assessment.

Behavioral Actions

_____
_____
_____
_____

Physical Actions

_____
_____
_____
_____

Emotional Actions

_____
_____
_____
_____

Cognitive Actions

_____
_____
_____
_____

Your Stress Management Style

How did your stress management style develop?

What factors influenced it?

Ways of Coping with Stress by Altering, Adapting and/or Avoiding the Stressor

- Seek to change the situation
- Be more organized
- Ask someone to alter his or her behavior
- Exercise
- Engage in deep breathing, meditation, etc.
- Be assertive
- Alter irrational beliefs
- Withdraw from the situation
- Accept the stressor
- Maintain good health by nurturing yourself

Tips for Coping with Stress

Changing old habits takes time. Do not attempt to change too much too soon or you might get frustrated.

Assess the types of support you will get from family and friends before choosing your coping strategies.

Remember that you cannot change or control everything. Focus on which you have control.

Do not expect a single coping strategy to "fix" the stressful situation.

SECTION II:
Physical Fitness Scale

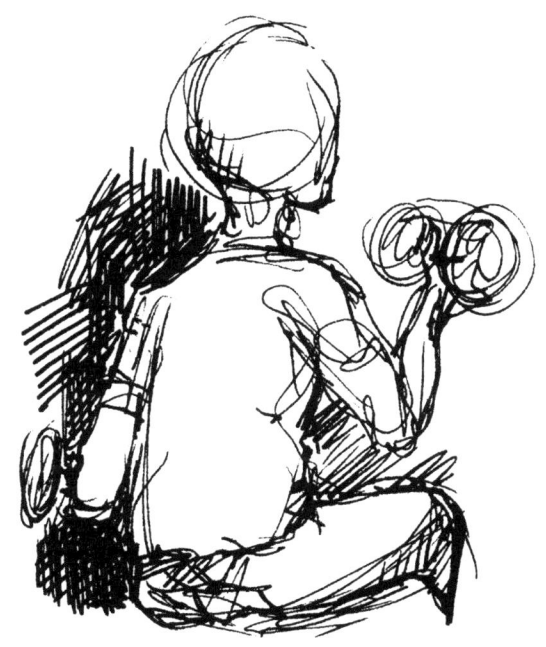

Name_____

Date_____

Physical Fitness Scale
Directions

We all need resources to meet the stressful demands posed by our environment. By taking responsibility for your health through regular exercise, good nutrition and rest, you will be physically fit, which will help you deal effectively with stress in your life.

This assessment contains 30 statements related to three important resistance resources that will help you build protection against your stress. Read each of the statements and decide whether or not the statement describes you. If the statement describes you, circle the number under the **YES** column next to that statement. If it does not describe you, circle the number under the **NO** column next to that statement.

In the following example, the circled number under **YES** indicates the statement is descriptive of the person completing the inventory.

	YES	NO
I. I think I get enough sleep every night	(2)	1

This is not a test and there are no right or wrong answers. Do not spend too much time thinking about your answers. Your initial response will likely be the most true for you. Be sure to respond to every statement.

(Turn to the next page and begin)

SECTION II: PHYSICAL FITNESS SCALE

Physical Fitness Scale

	YES	NO
I. I think I get enough sleep every night	2	1
I. I am rarely irritable from a lack of sleep	2	1
I. I have a regular sleep routine	2	1
I. I am frequently drowsy during the day	1	2
I. I can function well with fewer than eight hours of sleep per night	2	1
I. I have fallen asleep in school or at work	1	2
I. I feel fatigued a lot of the time	1	2
I. I will take short naps during the day if I need to	2	1
I. I have difficulty falling asleep	1	2
I. My partner keeps me awake at night	1	2
I. TOTAL	_____	_____
II. I do not keep myself fit	1	2
II. Taking care of my body is important to me	2	1
II. I make an effort to stay physically active	2	1
II. I am proud of how I look and feel	2	1
II. I don't exercise if I don't feel like it	1	2
II. I take time to exercise vigorously	2	1
II. I don't have time to exercise	1	2
II. I have a long-term exercise plan I stick to	2	1
II. I set aside a regular time for exercising	2	1
II. I use the proper equipment when I exercise	2	1
II. TOTAL	_____	_____

(Continued on the next page)

SECTION II: PHYSICAL FITNESS SCALE

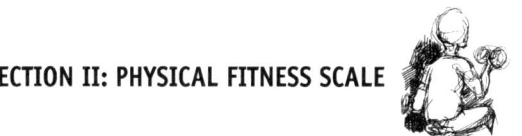

(Physical Fitness Scale, continued)

III. I maintain my appropriate weight	2	1
III. I eat lots of fresh fruits and vegetables	2	1
III. I have irregular and inconsistent eating habits	1	2
III. Whenever possible, I minimize salt (sodium) intake	2	1
III. I am conscious of my cholesterol and fat intake	2	1
III. In my diet I minimize foods that contain large amounts of sugar	2	1
III. I consume way too many calories	1	2
III. I do not eat a lot of "fast foods"	2	1
III. I often eat too much food at meals	1	2
III. I consume excess amounts of alcohol	1	2

III. TOTAL _____   _____

(Go to the Scoring Directions on the next page)

SECTION II: PHYSICAL FITNESS SCALE

Physical Fitness Scale Scoring Directions

This assessment is designed to help you explore if you are building up a protective reserve so when you encounter stress, you will be able to cope effectively. From the Physical Fitness Scale, add the numbers that you circled in Section I. This will allow you to get your Sleep score. You will get a total in the range from 10 to 20. Put that number in the space marked next to the Sleep Total below. Do the same for the other two scales: II – Exercise score, and III – Nutrition score. Then, transfer these totals to the spaces below:

I. Sleep Total   =   _____

II. Exercise Total   =   _____

III. Nutrition Total =   _____

To find your overall Physical Fitness total, you can add together the three scores above. Total scores range from 30 to 60. Put that score in the space below.

Physical Fitness TOTAL   =   _____

Profile Interpretation

Scores from 17 to 20 in any single area, or a total score from 51 to 60, are HIGH
and indicate that you are building the generalized resistance resources necessary to cope effectively with stress when you encounter it. Exercises on the following pages will help you to continue building resistance resources.

Scores from 14 to 16 in any single area, or a total score from 40 to 50, are AVERAGE
and indicate that you are building some of the generalized resistance resources necessary to cope effectively with stress when you encounter it. It would be helpful to do even more. Complete the exercises on the following pages to build the resistance resources you need to cope more effectively.

Scores from 10 and 13 in any single area, or a total score from 30 to 39, are LOW
and indicate that you are not yet building the generalized resistance resources necessary to cope effectively with stress when you encounter it. Complete the exercises on the following pages to build the resistance resources you need to cope more effectively.

SECTION II: ACTIVITY HANDOUTS

Building Resistance Resources

Coping effectively with stress is a skill that can be learned. You can build resistance resources to help you to promote health and well-being, and to serve as a shield against stress you encounter from your environment. Complete the following activities to build healthy buffers against stress.

Sleep

A major buffer that can ensure good physical health is adequate sleep. Sleep is critical for you to be able to rejuvenate both your body and your mind. Sleep deficiency can cause irritability, depression, anxiety, and many physical disorders. It is estimated that more than 100 million people work and engage in leisure activities without enough sleep. Some of the suggestions provided by sleep experts include the following:

Establish a sleep routine – Although you may lead a very busy life with family and social commitments, education and work, it is still very important to develop and follow a routine before you fall asleep. Some of the things people do include reading, watching a movie, or doing a puzzle.

What are your habits before bedtime? _____

_____

On average, how many hours of sleep do you get per night? _____

Do you feel this is the amount you need? Why or why not?_____

_____

What time do you go to bed at night? _____ Would there be a better time? _____

What keeps you from going to bed at that time? _____

_____

What time do you get up? What is your morning routine? _____

_____

_____

How much do you nap? When do you take naps? _____

_____

How do these naps help you? _____

_____

Things That Steal My Sleep

SLEEP STEALERS	HOW THEY STEAL MY SLEEP
Stress / Racing mind	
Alcohol / Substances	
Caffeine	
Eating habits	
Partner with sleep problems	
Distractions (TV, books, computers)	
Noise level	
Temperature	
Lighting	
Physical problems (arthritis, asthma, illness, etc.)	
Effects of medication	
Changing sleep times	
Lack of exercise	
New medication	
Other	

SECTION II: ACTIVITY HANDOUTS

Exercise

Physical activity and exercise are two of the most effective ways to lessen the effects of stress and to promote recovery more easily from stressful events. Research has shown that exercise can greatly reduce the effects of stress on your body. To maximize the stress-reduction benefits of regular exercise try the following:

1) Identify the best form of exercise for you.

What types of exercise do you get each day (jogging, walking, swimming, aerobics, etc.)?

_____
_____
_____

Which of these types of exercise do you enjoy most? Why?

_____
_____
_____

2) Monitor the overall amount of exercise you get.

How often do you engage in the above activities?

_____
_____
_____

What is the duration of time that you engage in the above activities?

_____
_____
_____

(Continued on the next page)

Exercise *(Continued)*

3) Evaluate the effectiveness of the exercise you get.

What types of physical effects do you notice when you are consistently exercising (better cardiovascular health, better sleep, faster recovery from stress, weight loss, increased energy, etc.)?

_____
_____
_____

What types of emotional effects do you notice when you are consistently exercising (mood stabilized, pent-up energy released, feelings of calm and well-being, etc.)?

_____
_____
_____

4) Look at other exercise options.

Have you found exercise classes you would like to take? What are they and where are they?

_____
_____
_____

Are there any team sports that you would like to get involved with?

_____
_____
_____

5) After answering the exercise questions and exploring exercise in your life, what are your thoughts, conclusions or goals?

_____
_____
_____
_____

Leisure-Time Physical Activity

Many people work at sedentary jobs, return home and engage in sedentary leisure-time activities like watching television, reading or using a computer. Leisure-time physical activity can be used to increase energy and reduce stress. Use the following table to identify those leisure-time activities that you are currently engaged in that can help you reduce stress. Examples of these leisure-time activities might include gardening, cutting grass, bowling, riding a bike, running, going out on a photo-hunt treasure or walking in the park.

BENEFITS TO MY HEALTH	MY LEISURE ACTIVITIES
Weight Control	*Example: I try and walk my dog every day. We walk around the neighborhood . . . probably about a half-mile per day.*
General Health	
Challenge	
Social Interaction	
Mental Challenge	
Stress Management	
Other	

SECTION II: ACTIVITY HANDOUTS

Setting Goals for Your Health

It is important for you to engage in physically active leisure activities and exercise to increase your overall health. This will help you to expend energy, reduce stress, and contribute to your healthy well-being. The following section will help you set goals for exercising and engaging in physically-active leisure activities. In the sections that follow, write both short-term goals (one to six months) and long-term goals (six months to a year into the future). Keep the following tips in mind as you set your goals:

Goal Setting

Set goals that include the following:

Time specific

List a date by which you will achieve the goal.

Personal

Set goals that apply to you. Do not worry about competing with other people. Do not let other people set goals for you. This is your health!

Written

Write your goals using the form that follows. Remember to change and update your goals as you need to.

Realistic

Set goals that you can achieve. Be realistic. If you set goals that are unachievable you will probably get frustrated and quit.

Measurable

Set goals that you can measure. For example, losing or gaining weight is not as measurable as losing or gaining five pounds in one month.

Revisable

Revise your goals periodically and set new or improved goals to keep you motivated.

SECTION II: ACTIVITY HANDOUTS

My Goals

Now it is time for you to set your own goals. In the table below, list some of your long-term goals and the short-term goals that will help you to reach your long-term goals. Remember to keep the suggestions outlined above in mind as you write your goals.

LONG-TERM GOALS	SHORT-TERM GOALS
Achieve my optimum body weight	- begin gardening every weekend, starting tomorrow - lose (or gain) about a pound a week, starting Monday - join a fitness center the 1st of next month

SECTION II: ACTIVITY HANDOUTS

Nutrition

Stress and nutrition are linked so that people who eat well tend to be more resilient to stressful situations, and yet most people tend to eat more and select a poor diet during time of stress. The following exercise is designed to help you examine your current diet.

NUTRITIOUS ELEMENTS	I EAT TOO MUCH OF THESE	I DO NOT EAT ENOUGH OF THESE
Proteins *(milk, eggs)*		
Fats *(butter, cheese)*		
Bad Carbohydrates *(sugar, soda)*		
Good Carbohydrates *(potatoes, fresh fruit)*		
Vitamins *(vegetables, fish)*		
Liquids *(water, tea)*		

My Physical Fitness

What have you learned about yourself in regard to your physical fitness?

_____
_____
_____
_____
_____
_____
_____
_____
_____
_____
_____
_____
_____
_____

What will you do to improve your physical fitness?

_____
_____
_____
_____
_____
_____
_____
_____
_____
_____
_____
_____
_____
_____

SECTION II: JOURNALING ACTIVITIES

My Physical Fitness Benefits

What benefits would you like to see within six months?

_____

What benefits would you like to see within one year?

_____

Eating Patterns and Links between Stress and Nutrition

- Eating junk food
- Munching all day long
- Eating too much before bedtime
- Not eating enough healthy foods
- Eating a lot of fast foods
- Eating too much
- Eating too little
- Alcohol and drug use
- Eating and drinking too much caffeine
- Consuming too much sugar

When you are starting an exercise program . . .

- Start slowly, add a little more each day

- Select aerobic activities you enjoy

- Put variety into your exercise regimen

- Set goals for yourself

- Set aside a regular time for exercising

- Exercise with friends if possible

- If you experience health problems, see a physician

SECTION III:
Creative Leisure Scale

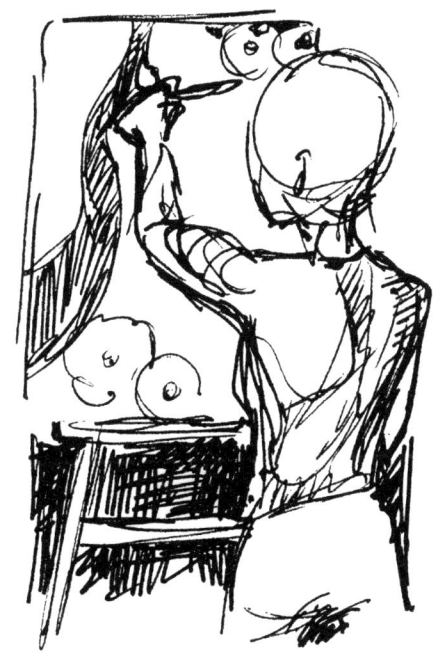

Name_____

Date_____

SECTION III: CREATIVE LEISURE SCALE

Creative Leisure Scale Directions

An important aspect of a wellness lifestyle is being able to find satisfying leisure activities to supplement or complement your life. Leisure interests are those interests that you pursue in your free time. These interests might include hobbies, recreational activities, family activities, volunteering, crafts, and sports. This assessment will help you identify possibilities that might appeal to you. It contains 63 statements divided into nine leisure interest categories. Read each statement carefully. Circle the number of the response that shows how descriptive each statement is of you. Answer all the questions using the following scale:

4 = Always   3 = Often   2 = Sometimes   1 = Rarely, if ever

In my spare time, I enjoy, or might enjoy . . .

1. attending art classes..4   (3)   2   1

Circling the number 3 indicates that the respondent often attends art classes or would like to attend them.

This is not a test and there are no right or wrong answers. Do not spend too much time thinking about your answers. Your initial response will likely be the most true for you. Be sure to respond to every statement.

(Turn to the next page and begin)

SECTION III: CREATIVE LEISURE SCALE

Creative Leisure

4 = Always   3 = Often   2 = Sometimes   1 = Rarely, if ever

In my spare time, I enjoy, or might enjoy . . .

1. attending art classes	4	3	2	1
2. drawing, painting or sculpting	4	3	2	1
3. going to a concert	4	3	2	1
4. writing poems or stories	4	3	2	1
5. using my skills in various arts and crafts	4	3	2	1
6. attending plays or musicals	4	3	2	1
7. sewing and needlecrafts	4	3	2	1

ARTS/CRAFTS = _____

In my spare time, I enjoy, or might enjoy . . .

8. activities that keep me fit and trim	4	3	2	1
9. training for marathons	4	3	2	1
10. walking to get or stay in shape	4	3	2	1
11. attending fitness and nutrition workshops	4	3	2	1
12. taking aerobics classes	4	3	2	1
13. weight lifting or martial arts	4	3	2	1
14. playing sports	4	3	2	1

HEALTH/FITNESS = _____

In my spare time, I enjoy, or might enjoy . . .

15. reading science books and magazines	4	3	2	1
16. looking through a microscope	4	3	2	1
17. visiting museums and/or historical sites	4	3	2	1
18. working mathematical games	4	3	2	1
19. gazing at the stars	4	3	2	1
20. predicting the weather	4	3	2	1
21. learning more about going into space	4	3	2	1

SCIENCE = _____

(Continued on the next page)

SECTION III: CREATIVE LEISURE SCALE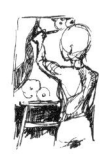

(Creative Leisure Scale, continued)

4 = Always   3 = Often   2 = Sometimes   1 = Rarely, if ever

In my spare time, I enjoy, or might enjoy . . .

22. helping other people	4	3	2	1
23. doing volunteer work	4	3	2	1
24. helping friends with personal problems	4	3	2	1
25. teaching	4	3	2	1
26. working with small children	4	3	2	1
27. helping people with disabilities	4	3	2	1
28. tutoring others	4	3	2	1

SOCIAL = _____

In my spare time, I enjoy, or might enjoy . . .

29. planning family recreational activities	4	3	2	1
30. cooking and baking	4	3	2	1
31. hosting parties at home	4	3	2	1
32. spending evenings at home with my family	4	3	2	1
33. driving members of my family to athletic events	4	3	2	1
34. cutting and styling hair for family members	4	3	2	1
35. vacationing with my family	4	3	2	1

HOME & FAMILY = _____

In my spare time, I enjoy, or might enjoy . . .

36. being in charge	4	3	2	1
37. holding office in clubs and organizations	4	3	2	1
38. organizing group activities	4	3	2	1
39. making decisions	4	3	2	1
40. working with finances	4	3	2	1
41. being responsible	4	3	2	1
42. planning activities for others	4	3	2	1

LEADING = _____

(Continued on the next page)

SECTION III: CREATIVE LEISURE SCALE

(Creative Leisure Scale, continued)

4 = Always   3 = Often   2 = Sometimes   1 = Rarely, if ever

In my spare time, I enjoy . . .

43. reading blueprints, manuals or maps	4	3	2	1
44. using hand tools	4	3	2	1
45. repairing computers	4	3	2	1
46. repairing cars	4	3	2	1
47. working with wood	4	3	2	1
48. operating heavy equipment	4	3	2	1
49. reading magazines about mechanical principles	4	3	2	1

MECHANICAL = _____

In my spare time, I enjoy . . .

50. playing with a domestic animal / pet	4	3	2	1
51. being on a farm	4	3	2	1
52. raising plants and flowers	4	3	2	1
53. landscaping yards	4	3	2	1
54. cutting grass and caring for lawns	4	3	2	1
55. caring for sick animals	4	3	2	1
56. planting and harvesting crops	4	3	2	1

PLANTS/ANIMALS = _____

In my spare time, I enjoy or might enjoy . . .

57. playing on my computer	4	3	2	1
58. having a massage	4	3	2	1
59. meditating	4	3	2	1
60. planting a vegetable or flower garden	4	3	2	1
61. going to a place of worship	4	3	2	1
62. reading a book	4	3	2	1
63. writing in my journal or diary	4	3	2	1

ALONE TIME = _____

(Go to the Scoring Directions on the next page)

SECTION III: CREATIVE LEISURE SCALE

Creative Leisure Scale Scoring Directions

The inventory you have just completed will help you identify various types of leisure activities that can help you reduce stress and enhance your life satisfaction. The assessment is designed to measure your leisure interests and help you identify leisure activities related to your interests. For each of the sections on the previous pages, add the scores you circled for each of the sections. Put that total on the line marked "Total" at the end of each section.

Then, transfer your totals to the spaces below:

TOTALS:

Arts/Crafts Scale _____

Health/Fitness Scale _____

Science Scale _____

Social Scale _____

Family Scale _____

Leading Scale _____

Mechanical Scale _____

Plants/Animals Scale _____

Alone Time Scale _____

After you have completed transferring your total scores, turn to the next page for the Profile Interpretation section with more information about your scores on the assessment.

SECTION III: CREATIVE LEISURE SCALE

Profile Interpretation

Use the information below to assist you in the interpretation of your scores.

If your score for any of the scales is 22 through 28, you probably have a great deal of interest in these types of leisure activities. If you have more than one score in this range, you might enjoy several different types of activities in your leisure time.

If your score for any of the scales is 14 to 21, you probably have some interest in these types of leisure activities. If your highest score falls in this range, activities on that scale will probably be the area in which you will find the most satisfying leisure–time enjoyment.

If your score for any of the scales is 7 through 13, you probably are not interested in these types of leisure activities.

Regardless of your score, the scale descriptions, exercises and activities that follow are designed to help you increase your leisure interests.

Scale Descriptions

1. ARTS / CRAFTS

People scoring high on this scale are interested in creatively expressing themselves through artistic endeavors. You need a way of expressing your feelings and ideas. You are creative, but you need a way to tap into your specific creative talents. Consider such leisure activities as painting, drawing, sketching, sculpting, photography, writing poems, ceramics, writing short stories, pottery, origami, reading, needlework, attending arts festivals, acting in community theatre, blogging, scrapbooking, designing web pages, taking dance lessons, singing in a choir or crafts.

2. HEALTH / FITNESS

People scoring high on this scale are interested in activities that are physically challenging and help to keep them physically fit. Engaging in physical activities is the best way for you to reduce your tension and anxiety. Consider such leisure activities as tennis, running in marathons, throwing darts, martial arts, chopping wood, yoga, mountain climbing, kayaking, scuba diving, rock–wall climbing, searching for buried treasure, coaching children's athletic games, amateur sports, weight lifting, health clubs, exercising, jogging, aerobics, softball, pilates, skiing, bowling, swimming, traveling, cycling, mall walking or canoeing.

(Continued on the next page)

SECTION III: CREATIVE LEISURE SCALE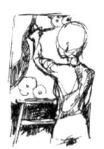

(Scale Descriptions, continued)

3. SCIENCE

People scoring high on this scale are interested in discovering, collecting, and analyzing information about the natural world, life sciences, and human behavior. Consider such leisure activities as astronomy, science fairs, health care volunteer, building model rockets, mathematical puzzles, amateur archeology, meteorology, star gazing, collecting rocks, exploring caves, weather watching, reading about technological developments, visiting planetariums and science museums, computer games, studying anatomy, prospecting, conducting experiments with plants, doing chemistry experiments, or watching aerospace shows on television or at an air show.

4. SOCIAL

People scoring high on this scale are interested in improving people's social, mental, emotional, and spiritual well–being. You feel a need to give back to other people and perhaps want to feel appreciated. Consider volunteering your time to help others in such leisure activities as tutoring others, helping the elderly, assisting the disabled, helping in a hospital, participation in religious and/or spiritual groups, dances, serving in a homeless shelter, babysitting, caring for children, visiting friends, going to parties, entertaining, going to amusement parks, becoming a mental health volunteer or teaching English as a second language.

5. FAMILY

People scoring high on this scale are interested in activities which allow them to be with other members of their family, significant others, or with friends. Consider such leisure activities as baking pastries, cake decorating, hosting parties, sewing, cooking, cutting hair for family members, planning family recreational activities, traveling with family members, shopping, taking children to school and/or athletic activities, watching sports, handling equipment for a local athletic team, serving family meals, teaching others how to cook or bake, canning and preserving food, or cooking for community events.

6. LEADING

People scoring high on this scale are interested in directing and leading other people. You enjoy being in charge and coordinating events. Consider such leisure activities as being an officer in an organization, coaching, organizing neighborhood activities, coordinating community events, holding public office, serving as a school board member, fund raising, working on an urban planning committee, becoming a scout leader, studying financial trends, organizing an investment group, campaigning for political endeavors, coordinating a camping trip, organizing religious events, being in charge of a community group, or arranging family activities.

(Continued on the next page)

SECTION III: CREATIVE LEISURE SCALE

(Scale Descriptions, continued)

7. MECHANICAL

People scoring high on this scale enjoy working with their hands and working with tools. You enjoy working with machines. Consider such leisure activities as fixing appliances, repairing computers, woodworking, home repairs, painting, repairing cars, auto body repair, wood carving, metal work, repairing watches and clocks, furniture repair, upholstery, model railroading, building cabinets, refurbishing antiques, plumbing, working on heating and air conditioners, reading blueprints, building houses for Habitat for Humanity, rebuilding old cars, watching home repair shows on television, or welding.

8. PLANTS/ANIMALS

People scoring high on this scale enjoy working to help, watch, or care for animals and study and grow plants. You enjoy "getting your hands dirty" and being with nature. You probably will enjoy such leisure activities as bird watching, riding horses, showing dogs, grooming animals, farming, reading about plants, going on hikes, taking nature walks, volunteering in a veterinarian's office, volunteering at an animal shelter, hunting, fishing, camping, visiting state parks, flower arranging, animal breeding, pet boarding, growing house plants, gardening, playing with pets, or landscaping.

9. ALONE TIME

People scoring high on this scale enjoy spending time engaging in leisure activities they can do by themselves. You probably are drawn to activities which allow you to connect with your spirituality. Consider such leisure activities as playing computer games, working on crossword puzzles, meditating, yoga, taking long walks, attending a retreat, camping, playing with a pet, doing a jigsaw puzzle, visiting museums, writing a book, driving on country roads, jogging, watching the sun set, hanging out in a bookstore, baking, reading in a coffee shop or gazing at the stars.

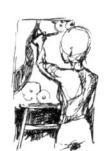

The Importance of Leisure

Leisure can be defined as a period of time that we have outside of work and essential household and relationship activities. The typical American employee spends about eight to ten hours a day working, five days a week. This totals at least forty to fifty hours per week. Most of us also spend a lot of time for compulsory activities such as eating, sleeping and essential chores. With the time left over, it is important for us to engage in leisure-time activities that will allow us to balance work, find enjoyment, and expend mental, physical, social and creative energy.

Leisure-time activities are usually more fun than work. We usually do not engage in leisure activities that we do not like to do. We often forget that it's all right to have fun. Many of us are workaholics who feel guilty when we take time for ourselves to enjoy fun activities. We do not want to take time away from our family, friends or obligations. But we can creatively incorporate time with family and friends and engage in leisure activities at the same time.

The skills you gain from leisure-time activities can easily be transferred to occupations. People are typically good at what they enjoy, are more motivated to participate in these activities, and will spend more time at them. Leisure-time activities can be valuable exploratory experiences in which individuals can develop both personal and work-related skills that might be useful in many different types of jobs. Similarly, leisure-time activities also provide an opportunity to expand and perfect skills you already have.

Most people work a lot of hours and work very hard. Although a certain amount of work is very good for us, it does not mean that twice as much work means that you get twice as much done. In fact, research indicates that the law of diminishing returns takes over and that you actually gain less and less for each extra hour that you work. In Japan, they have a term, Karoshi, which means sudden death from overwork. Leisure can help you to remain balanced.

Ernie Zelenski, in his book, *The Joy of Not Working*, suggests that when people are able to enjoy leisure time to the fullest, their lives will be enhanced to immeasurable levels. Some of the benefits people enjoy from satisfying leisure include:

- A higher quality of life
- Personal growth
- Improved health
- Higher self-esteem
- Less stress
- A more relaxed lifestyle
- Excitement and adventure
- A balanced lifestyle
- A sense of self-worth
- An increase in quality of family life

Developmental Leisure Exercise

Think about what you like to do in your spare time for fun and relaxation. Do you enjoy physical activities such as jogging, bowling, or weight lifting; do you enjoy creative activities such as writing poetry, dancing, or painting pictures; maybe you enjoy helping others by volunteering at the local hospital, tutoring others, or caring for sick friends and relatives; or would you rather engage in scientific leisure activities such as weather watching, amateur archeology, or astronomy. These are just a few different types of leisure activities. There are many more which you might enjoy. Throughout your life, what have been your favorite leisure activities and what was happening in your life that steered you toward these particular leisure activities? For example, you may have started studying the stars because you had a great astronomy class in college. List and include all of your past leisure activities below, in which you participated.

Age	Activities	What was happening in my life
0–10	*Example: Roller Skating*	*Living with my mom and roller skating every night before dinner with my friend Gerta.*
11–20		
21–30		
31–40		
41–50		
51–60		
61–70		
71+		

SECTION III: ACTIVITY HANDOUTS

Leisure Exploration

Answer the following questions to help you further explore the responses that you provided in the previous exercise:

1. What leisure activity feels good to you now? Is there a similar occupation that would use that activity or skill?

   _____
   _____
   _____

2. What activity has brought you the most joy over the past five years?

   _____
   _____
   _____

3. What type of personality characteristics do you have, and what leisure activities are best suited to your personality?

   _____
   _____
   _____

4. Which leisure activity do you really look forward to doing?

   _____
   _____
   _____

5. What type of leisure activities would give you the emotional rewards you want?

   _____
   _____
   _____

6. Which leisure activities would be good to do when you're feeling stressed?

   _____
   _____
   _____

SECTION III: ACTIVITY HANDOUTS

Overcoming Barriers to Leisure Participation

Barriers are conditions that stand in your way of participating in your favorite leisure activities or from participating as often as you would like. Many different reasons set up barriers. There are times when you may want to do something and you are unable to engage in the leisure activity. You may have a variety of reasons to justify your inability to participate in your favorite leisure activities.

I. Money

Lack of money could be a barrier to your leisure participation. Because many leisure activities cost money, you might lack the financial resources required to participate in and enjoy your leisure interests.

How has lack of money stopped you from engaging in leisure activities?

_____

_____

_____

_____

II. Free Time

Lack of free time could be a barrier to your leisure participation. This barrier involves not having enough time or not taking advantage of the time you do have.

Describe how you often have trouble finding the time to engage in your favorite leisure activities? How can you solve this issue?

_____

_____

_____

_____

(Continued on the next page)

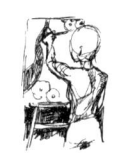

SECTION III: ACTIVITY HANDOUTS

(Overcoming Barriers to Leisure Participation, continued)

III. Availability

Lack of availability could be a barrier to your leisure participation. Perhaps there are times when you would like to participate in a leisure activity but cannot because you do not have adequate transportation, the activity or program is not available in your community, your work schedule interferes, or physical barriers may exist.

What types of activities are unavailable to you?

_____
_____
_____

Why are these activities unavailable to you and how could you find a way to make them or others like them available?

_____
_____
_____

IV. Health

Your health might be a barrier to your leisure participation. Your health may sometimes inhibit your participation in leisure activities. You may have physical or mental disabilities that prevent you from concentrating on and/or participating in recreational activities.

What health barriers have you had? Which barriers do you still have today?

_____
_____
_____

Which activities could you engage in, despite these barriers.

_____
_____
_____

Leisure Activities

How do you think leisure activities can help you in your relationships?

_____
_____
_____
_____
_____

How do you think leisure activities can help you in your social life?

_____
_____
_____
_____
_____

How do you think leisure activities can help you in your job or career?

_____
_____
_____
_____
_____

How do you think leisure activities can help you with your self-satisfaction?

_____
_____
_____
_____
_____

Characteristics of Leisure

- Leisure involves the use of time outside of work, chores and obligations.

- Leisure time is time free from the need to play other roles, such as those of student, employee, homemaker, family member and citizen.

- Leisure time may, as in playing tennis, require the expenditure of effort, or it may, as in relaxing in a hammock, require no effort.

- Leisure pursuits are often engaged in to meet some personal needs, support values, and use abilities.

- A leisure activity may have clear goals, such as creating a painting, or they can be something like just relaxing.

- Leisure activities may support, conflict with, or be neutral to one's other roles, in their use of time and effort.

SECTION IV:
Healthy Relationships Scale

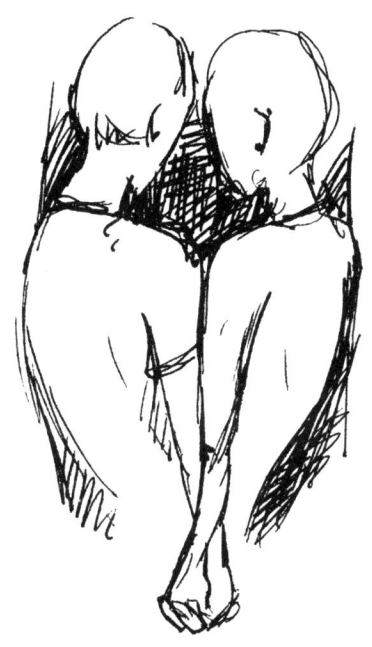

Name_____

Date_____

SECTION IV: HEALTHY RELATIONSHIPS SCALE

Healthy Relationships Scale Directions

Healthy intimate relationships are critical in helping you to live a wellness lifestyle. Although a healthy relationship takes time and work, when a healthy intimate relationship is achieved, you will feel secure and satisfied whether you are with your partner or not. People in a healthy intimate relationship experience intellectual, emotional, and physical intimacy. The purpose of this assessment is to help you identify if you are in a healthy intimate relationship and if not, how you and your partner can become more intimate.

This booklet contains 24 statements divided into three sections. Read each statement and decide how true the statement is for you. In the following example, the circled 2 indicates that the statement is **Somewhat True** for the person completing the inventory:

3 = True **2 = Somewhat True** **1 = Not True**

SECTION I: INTELLECTUAL INTIMACY

I share my most private thoughts with my partner   3   (2)   1

This is not a test and there are no right or wrong answers. Do not spend too much time thinking about your answers. Your initial response will likely be the most true for you. Be sure to respond to every statement.

(Turn to the next page and begin)

SECTION IV: HEALTHY RELATIONSHIPS SCALE

Healthy Relationships Scale

3 = True   2 = Somewhat True   1 = Not True

SECTION I: INTELLECTUAL INTIMACY

I share most of my private thoughts with my partner	3	2	1
I feel like I can trust my partner when I share intimate information	3	2	1
I often bounce ideas off of my partner for a second opinion	3	2	1
I am able to communicate my dreams to my partner	3	2	1
I feel comfortable sharing my most intimate needs with my partner	3	2	1
I often tell my partner about my life and career desires	3	2	1
I often talk with my partner about our future together	3	2	1
I feel a deep connection with my partner	3	2	1

TOTAL = _____

SECTION II: EMOTIONAL INTIMACY

I am able to connect on a feeling level with my partner	3	2	1
I am able to communicate my feelings of love	3	2	1
I am able to express my feelings when I am angry	3	2	1
I am able to express my feelings in an unguarded way	3	2	1
My partner constructively receives the expression of my feelings	3	2	1
I am emotionally close with my partner	3	2	1
I am not afraid to express my feelings at any time	3	2	1
I trust my partner enough to tell him/her almost anything	3	2	1

TOTAL = _____

(Continued on the next page)

SECTION IV: HEALTHY RELATIONSHIPS SCALE

(Healthy Relationships Scale, continued)

3 = True **2 = Somewhat True** **1 = Not True**

SECTION III: PHYSICAL INTIMACY

I have a physically intimate relationship with my partner	3	2	1
I often hug my significant other to show support	3	2	1
I often touch my significant other when it is needed	3	2	1
I will hold my partner's hand in public	3	2	1
I show my deep love for my partner through sexual intimacy	3	2	1
I know, and I accept, when my partner needs time to be alone	3	2	1
I give my partner special attention and receive it from him/her	3	2	1
My partner is physically intimate with me	3	2	1

TOTAL = _____

(Go to the Scoring Directions on the next page)

SECTION IV: HEALTHY RELATIONSHIPS SCALE

Healthy Relationships Scale
Scoring Directions

Being in an intimate relationship can be one of the greatest sources of human joy. Relationships that endure and deepen are formed by partners who share intellectual, emotional, and physical intimacy. Add the scores for each section and write the totals below.

SECTION I TOTAL = _____ (Intellectual Intimacy)

SECTION II TOTAL = _____ (Emotional Intimacy)

SECTION III TOTAL = _____ (Physical Intimacy)

Profile Interpretation

Individual Scale Score	Result	Indications
19 to 24	high	Your relationship has many of the characteristics and qualities explored on this scale. Continue to work at your relationship to keep it intellectually, emotionally, and physically intimate.
14 to 18	moderate	Your relationship has some of the characteristics and qualities explored on this scale. It would be helpful to develop additional skills and characteristics needed in order to have a healthier intimate relationship.
8 to 13	low	Your relationship has a few of the characteristics and qualities explored on this scale. It is important to further develop the skills and characteristics in order to have a healthy intimate relationship.

The higher your score on the scales of this assessment, the more intimate your relationship is. In the areas in which you score in the **Moderate** or **Low** range, make efforts to ensure that you continue to work at your relationship to make it more intimate. No matter if you scored **Low**, **Moderate** or **High**, the exercises and activities that follow are designed to help you to develop a more intimate relationship with your partner.

ID: 1
Exercises for Relationship Enhancement

Partner Exploration

The more you know about each other's inner worlds, the more profound the relationship between you and your partner will be. Self-exploration and the sharing of this exploration with your partner will have exciting and lasting effects on your relationship.

The following questions are designed to guide you and your partner through the self-exploration process and then to help each of you share this information with one another. Answer the following questions separately, as truthfully as possible, and then discuss your entries with each other.

What do you love best about your partner?

_____
_____
_____
_____
_____
_____
_____

What do you wish you could tell your partner but have neglected to do so?

_____
_____
_____
_____
_____
_____
_____

What does your partner do that annoys you the most?

_____
_____
_____
_____
_____
_____
_____

Appreciation

Showing appreciation for your partner is critical in building and maintaining an effective relationship. Complete the following statements listed below:

I appreciate the following characteristics about my partner…

_____
_____
_____
_____
_____

I appreciate the way my partner…

_____
_____
_____
_____
_____

I appreciate the way my partner handled the following situation…

_____
_____
_____
_____
_____

I appreciate my partner for…

_____
_____
_____
_____
_____

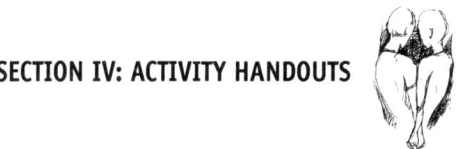

SECTION IV: ACTIVITY HANDOUTS

Relationship Philosophy

Each couple brings a different philosophy to their relationship. This philosophy comes from personality traits, parental role models, and childhood history. Answer the following questions to learn more about your relationship philosophy and that of your significant other:

Why do you think relationships work effectively?
_____
_____

Why do you think that relationships fail?
_____
_____

What was your parent's relationship like? Describe different aspects of this relationship.
_____
_____

What do you remember about the first year of your current relationship?
_____
_____

How is your relationship different now from when you first met?
_____
_____

Why did you and your partner become a couple?
_____
_____

What are your beliefs about children in your relationship?
_____
_____

What are your beliefs about careers in your relationship?
_____
_____

Conflict

Conflict occurs in all relationships. Think about how you and your partner handle conflict in your relationship. Think about your last disagreement or argument.

What were you arguing about (finances, hopes, children, fears, etc.)?

_____
_____
_____

What triggered the argument?

_____
_____
_____

What was the outcome of this argument?

_____
_____

What feelings were expressed in this argument?

_____
_____

What was your contribution to the argument?

_____
_____
_____

How could you avoid this type of argument in the future?

_____
_____
_____

What could your partner do to avoid this type of argument in the future?

_____
_____
_____

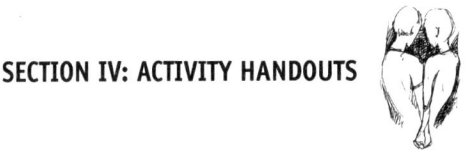

SECTION IV: ACTIVITY HANDOUTS

Sending Emotional Messages

In effective relationships, partners are able to express themselves by sending their partner emotional messages. Complete the following statements to think about the emotional messages you would like to send to your partner.

I get scared when you . . .

_____
_____
_____
_____
_____
_____

You hurt my feelings when you . . .

_____
_____
_____
_____
_____
_____

I feel unappreciated when you . . .

_____
_____
_____
_____
_____

I am sad when you . . .

_____
_____
_____
_____
_____

(Continued on the next page)

SECTION IV: ACTIVITY HANDOUTS

(Sending Emotional Messages, continued)

I disagree with you about . . .

_____
_____
_____
_____

I am thankful that you . . .

_____
_____
_____
_____
_____
_____

I love when you . . .

_____
_____
_____
_____
_____
_____

I want you to be more . . .

_____
_____
_____
_____
_____

I get excited when you . . .

_____
_____
_____
_____
_____

Family and/or Friend Issues

Most partners in an intimate relationship bring some sort of family and/or friend issues to the union. The following exercise will help you to identify those issues and develop a plan for developing effective coping skills.

Describe your relationship with your partner's family and/or friends.
_____
_____
_____
_____

On what issues is your partner not on your side?
_____
_____
_____
_____

On what issues are you not on your partner's side?
_____
_____
_____
_____

Describe how you would like your partner to treat your family and/or friends.
_____
_____
_____
_____

Describe how your partner would like you to treat his/her family and/or friends.
_____
_____
_____
_____

Finances

The use of finances and financial planning can be a major issue in most relationships. Confronting significant money conflicts is critical in the health of your relationship.

Complete the following exercises to determine how much of a problem money is in your intimate relationships.

Have you and your partner set-up a financial plan? Describe it.

_____
_____
_____

How would you describe your considerations about money?

_____
_____

How would you describe your partner's considerations about money?

_____
_____

How do you wish your partner would spend and save money?

_____
_____

How does your partner wish you would spend and save money?

_____
_____

What are your long-term financial goals?

_____
_____
_____

What can your partner do to help in meeting this goal?

_____
_____
_____

Techniques

Some problem-solving techniques *I have used* with my partner . . .

New Techniques

Some problem-solving techniques I would like to try with my partner . . .

Qualities of a Healthy Relationship

- **Enthusiasm for the relationship**

- **Acceptance of differences**

- **Appreciation for each other**

- **Support for one another**

- **Loyalty to each other**

- **Active listening to each other**

- **Love for each other**

- **Trust for each other**

- **Healthy communications**

SECTION V:
Spiritual Wellness Scale

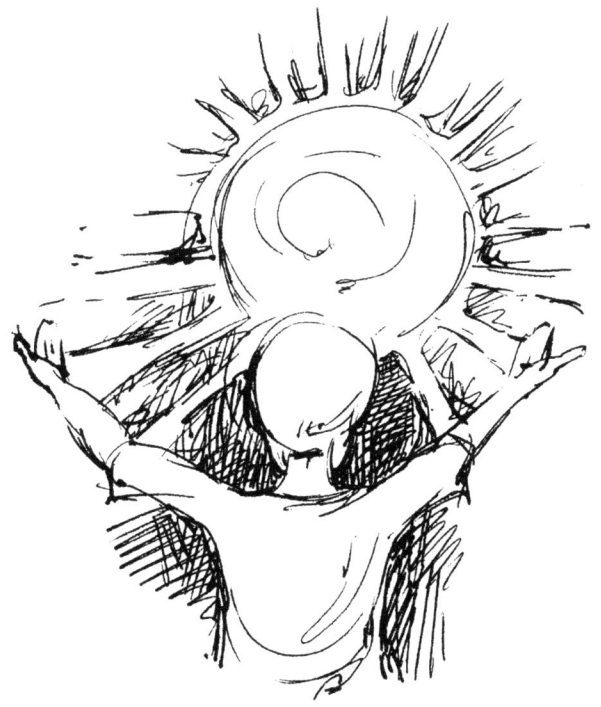

Name_____

Date_____

SECTION V: SPIRITUAL WELLNESS SCALE

Spiritual Wellness Scale Directions

Spiritual wellness is very important in your overall well-being. The spiritually well person is moved toward meaningful identity and purpose. It is a commitment to a worthwhile cause, purpose, and faith. The spiritually well person develops the inner Self and explores a personal purpose for life. Spiritual wellness is present when you are able to explore, identify, and implement a plan related to your life purpose. The Spiritual Wellness Inventory can help you to identify how you are experiencing spiritual well-being in your life.

The following assessment contains 32 statements. Use the choices listed below. Read each of the statements and circle the number to the right that best describes how much you value each statement.

>Circle **4** if the statement is **Very True** for you
>
>Circle **3** if the statement is **True** for you
>
>Circle **2** if the statement is **Somewhat True** for you
>
>Circle **1** if the statement is **Not True** for you

In the following example, the circled "3" indicates that the statement is True for the person completing the inventory:

ACTIVITY	**RESPONSE**
I know what my true purpose is	4　(3)　2　1

This is not a test and there are no right or wrong answers. Do not spend too much time thinking about your answers. Your initial response will likely be the most true for you. Be sure to respond to every statement.

(Turn to the next page and begin)

SECTION V: SPIRITUAL WELLNESS SCALE

Spiritual Wellness Scale

	VERY TRUE	TRUE	SOMEWHAT TRUE	NOT TRUE
I know what my true purpose is	4	3	2	1
I seek experiences which bring new meaning	4	3	2	1
I realize that there is a reason to live for the future	4	3	2	1
I have unique personally meaningful experiences	4	3	2	1
I have experiences which lead toward growth	4	3	2	1
I am continually searching for meaning and purpose	4	3	2	1
I seek ways challenge my full potential	4	3	2	1
I work to develop my inner self	4	3	2	1

MEANING & PURPOSE TOTAL _____

	VERY TRUE	TRUE	SOMEWHAT TRUE	NOT TRUE
I want to do something worthwhile for others	4	3	2	1
I do things without thinking, "What's in it for me?"	4	3	2	1
I try to understand the connectedness of people and things	4	3	2	1
I feel good when I cause someone to smile	4	3	2	1
I want to contribute to my community	4	3	2	1
I like contributing to the well being of others	4	3	2	1
I enjoy doing volunteer work	4	3	2	1
I feel a spiritual connection to other people	4	3	2	1

ALTRUISM TOTAL _____

(Continued on the next page)

SECTION V: SPIRITUAL WELLNESS SCALE

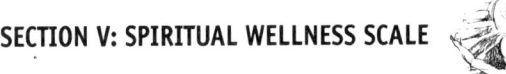

(Spiritual Wellness Scale, continued)

	VERY TRUE	TRUE	SOMEWHAT TRUE	NOT TRUE
I am aware of a force greater than myself	4	3	2	1
I am conscious of a greater power in my daily activities	4	3	2	1
I spend some time each day in prayer, meditation, or reflective thought	4	3	2	1
I am able to deal with stress because of my belief system	4	3	2	1
I consider myself spiritual or religious	4	3	2	1
I have specific spiritual or religious beliefs	4	3	2	1
I have faith in a higher power	4	3	2	1
I believe in a power that brings all of humanity together	4	3	2	1

HIGHER POWER TOTAL _____

	VERY TRUE	TRUE	SOMEWHAT TRUE	NOT TRUE
I am able to experience peace and balance in my life	4	3	2	1
I am content and do not look to external sources for happiness	4	3	2	1
I enjoy being with people different from me	4	3	2	1
When I am frustrated or sad, my spiritual beliefs give me direction	4	3	2	1
I am optimistic and rarely give up hope	4	3	2	1
I experience a sense of awe about my life	4	3	2	1
I experience playful moments daily	4	3	2	1
I see every life as sacred	4	3	2	1

CONTENTMENT TOTAL _____

(Go to the Scoring Directions on the next page)

SECTION V: SPIRITUAL WELLNESS SCALE

Spiritual Wellness Scale
Scoring Directions

Spiritual wellness is an important factor in your overall health and general well being. For each of the four sections on the previous pages, add the scores you circled. Put that total on the line marked "Total" at the end of each section.

Then, transfer your totals to the spaces below:

MEANING & PURPOSE TOTAL = _____

ALTRUISM TOTAL = _____

HIGHER POWER TOTAL = _____

SPIRITUAL VIRTUES TOTAL = _____

Profile Interpretation

Total Scales Score	Result	Indications
25 to 32	high	You are investing the time and energy in your spirituality and doing the things you need to do in order to experience spiritual growth.
16 to 24	moderate	You are investing some time and energy in your spirituality and doing some of the things you need to do in order to experience spiritual growth.
8 to 15	low	You are rarely investing the time and energy in your spirituality and/or doing the things you need to do in order to experience spiritual growth.

For scales which you scored in the **Moderate** or **High** range, find the descriptions on the pages that follow. Then, read the description and complete the exercises that are included. No matter how you scored, low, moderate or high, you will benefit from these exercises.

Spiritual Wellness Scale Descriptions

Meaning and Purpose

People scoring high on this scale have the sense that their life is meaningful, purposeful, and directed toward some greater good. Spiritual wellness provides that sense because it comprises the ethics, values, and morals that guide behavior and decisions, gives life meaning and provides direction for life. Optimal spiritual wellness occurs when people are able to discover, articulate, and then put that purpose to work in their life.

Altruism

People scoring high on this scale are able to find self-fulfillment through contributing to others' well-being. It is a selfless concern for other people. When they are altruistic, they are motivated to help others or do good acts, even though they do not receive a reward for it. It is giving without regard to reward or recognition and is a sincere desire to help others or sacrifice for the benefit of others.

Higher Power

People scoring high on this scale tend to believe in a higher power. They are open to the universal truths and the varied human experience of a power greater than themselves. They have their own conception of that greater power. This conception is based on their own images and/ or experiences. Whether this conception is part of an organized religion or simply a symbol that points to some aspects of spiritual maturity, their belief becomes a framework that guides decisions, and cushions and strengthens them to meet disappointments in their life.

Spiritual Virtues

People scoring high on this scale are able to apply spiritual practices in their daily life. They are able to embody and practice faith, optimism, and hope that sustains people through whatever life has to offer. They are working to develop their inner resources and identify a deep purpose to life that actually occurs when they are finally able to effectively discover, articulate, and act on purpose. They tend to be content with their lives, and are able to find harmony between what lies within them and the social and physical pressures outside of them.

Spiritual Wellness Exercises

Following are some general exercises designed to help you enhance your spiritual awareness and spiritual wellness.

Spiritual Meditation

Take time for your spiritual self. During this time, focus on the positive aspects of yourself, your family members, and the universe. You may choose to focus on a particular aspect every day that is important to you. For example, one day you may want to focus on peace throughout the world, while on the next day you might focus on the health of your family and yourself. Plan to spend thirty minutes, two or three times a week to start. Then you can expand your practice as you begin to grow spiritually. Do not let negative thoughts come into your mind. When you begin to think negative thoughts, stop them and replace them with more positive thoughts.

Spiritual Writing

In addition to the writing you are doing in this chapter, you may want to start a spirituality journal. In this journal you can focus on and write about your spiritual experiences on your journey. Writing daily about spiritual subjects can enhance your spiritual wellness. Begin by writing the date at the top of the page. Then write a brief sentence to describe the events of your day. After you have done this, you should then take time to reflect on the events from a spiritual perspective. Include anything that seems relevant or important in your life and your spirituality. Do not judge the content of your writing, just let it flow. Now, try it for today:

Date_____

Events of the day_____
_____
_____
_____
_____
_____

My spiritual perspective_____
_____
_____
_____
_____
_____

SECTION V: ACTIVITY HANDOUTS

Life Purpose

Purpose has been described as the recognition of the presence of the sacred within us and the choice of activities that are consistent with that presence. Purpose is equivalent to our contribution to life and humanity. Purpose may find expression through family, community, relationships, work, and spiritual activities. We receive from life what we give, and in the process we understand more of what it means to discover our purpose.

Discovering your purpose in life is the most important discovery of your life. Each person has a different, very natural reason for being. Purpose is the reason each person is born.

Why do you think you were born?

_____
_____
_____
_____

You are on your own quest to identify your purpose. A purpose adds meaning to our lives. Most people spend a lifetime attempting to identify their true purpose. At this point in your life, what do you think is your true purpose?

_____
_____
_____
_____

In what ways have you fulfilled – or begun to fulfill – that purpose?

_____
_____
_____
_____

If you feel you have not fulfilled – begun to fulfill – that purpose, what is keeping you from doing so?

_____
_____
_____
_____

(Life Purpose continued on the next page)

Life Purpose *(Continued)*

Purpose is that dimension of our spirit which is core to our being. It is who we are, why we are here, and where we are going. These are the three existential questions that must be answered for us to determine our purpose. Purpose is our life direction and source of essence.

Purpose is not simply finding out what your interests are or what job you are best suited for. It is much more. It is finding out who we are based on our life with our family, other relationships, work and leisure choices. By identifying our true purpose, we are able to transcend our daily needs. Defining our true purpose is a truly spiritual mission. Deep within our soul lies our purpose. We all contribute to life in a very unique fashion. Dig down deep and respond to the questions based on your core spiritual being; don't give surface answers (I am Jane Smith, etc.).

Life's Existential Questions	My Existential Answers
Who am I?	
Why am I here?	
Where am I going?	

Discovering Your Purpose

Purpose helps you to create a larger meaning in your life by feeding five deep, spiritual hungers:

1. Connecting with the creative spirit of life

What types of creative things do you do that bring you joy?

_____
_____
_____

2. Actively discovering and expressing our gifts

What are your gifts and how do you express them?

_____
_____
_____

3. Knowing that our life has made a difference

What could you do to ensure that your life has made a difference?

_____
_____
_____

4. Committing to something larger than yourself

Look beyond your most immediate needs and define some cause or purpose larger than your own success that gives you a sense of purpose. What is that cause or purpose?

_____
_____
_____

5. Feeling a sense of joy

Purpose helps people feel a sense of joy in life, and that the one constant factor in the daily lives of people who experience life satisfaction is the discovery of their purpose. What helps you to feel a sense of joy in life?

_____
_____
_____

SECTION V: ACTIVITY HANDOUTS

Forgiveness

Forgiveness is essential for spiritual wellness. Forgiveness is the ability to accept the core of all people and give them and yourself the gift of not being judgmental. Learning to forgive others is much easier than you think, but it requires practice. Continue writing on the reverse side of this paper if you need more space.

1. Start small. Think about some things that have happened to you and the people you would like to forgive. Who are they and for what could you forgive them?

_____
_____
_____

2. Postpone judgment. Think about the different ways that you judge other people? What patterns can you identify?

_____
_____
_____

3. Forgive and accept. Think about the people in your life that you would like to forgive (this may include yourself). Now forgive them in the spaces that follow:

Person I could forgive	For what I am forgiving them
My father	*I forgive my father for spending most of my childhood working long hours. I now know that he was trying to provide for me and my brother.*

Spend Time in Nature

You can experience your presence in the natural world by spending solitary time in a natural setting. Some of the activities that would enhance your spiritual wellness might include watching the sun set, listening to the waves hit against the shore, feeling a breeze on your face, listening to the rain fall on the roof of your house or lying in a field of grass. What are some things you might do in order to connect or reconnect with nature?

_____
_____
_____
_____

Express Your Creativity

You should begin to set aside time during your day to express your creative side. This time might be spent singing, writing, decorating, or painting. What do you enjoy that would allow you to express your creative side?

_____
_____
_____
_____

Engage in Spiritual Practice

You can practice activities that allow you to tune out the outer world and turn your attention inward, focusing on spiritual experiences. What do you enjoy that would allow you to focus inward (prayer, meditation, yoga, chanting, etc.)?

_____
_____
_____
_____

Perform Community Service

Volunteering allows you to foster a sense of community and a feeling of altruism. Some examples of community service might include volunteering at a clothing bank or food bank, mentoring children, working for a literacy project or visiting seniors in a retirement facility. Where are you volunteering and where might you like to volunteer?

I am currently volunteering at _____

I would like to volunteer at _____

Family Influences

When you were growing up, how did your family life influence your spiritually?

Spiritual Practices

What spiritual practices do you intend to work on to enhance your wellness?

Qualities of Spirituality

- **Having hope**

- **Appreciating differences in others**

- **Being non-judgmental**

- **Trusting your intuition**

- **Questioning nature**

- **Experiencing joy**

- **Developing a code of living**

- **Using moral reasoning**

- **Accepting ambiguity and mystery**

- **Forgiving yourself and others**

BONUS SECTION:
Life Skills Scale

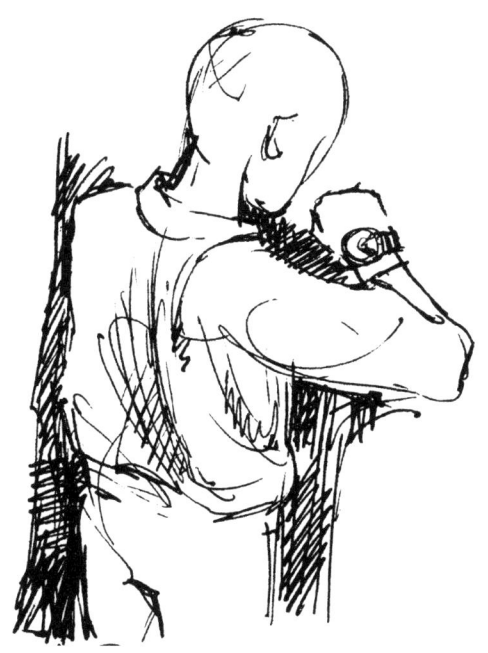

Name_____

Date_____

SECTION VI: LIFE SKILLS SCALE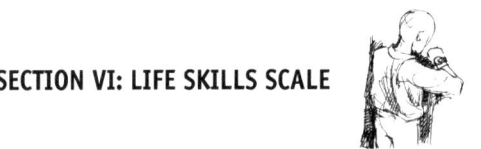

Life Skills Scale Directions

Current thinking in modern psychology suggests that the ability to manage daily life skills may actually be more important than having a high IQ. Life skills are those critical skills which help you to be healthy, productive, and to reach your full potential. Life skills are also vital survival skills people need for personal and career development. They help you deal more effectively with your environment and the people in that environment. Life skills, unlike the knowledge measured by traditional Intelligence Quotient (IQ) tests, are skills that can be learned or refined so that you can lead a successful, satisfying and productive life.

This scale contains 48 statements that are divided into four life skill categories. Read each of the statements and decide whether or not the statement describes you. Circle the number to the right of each statement that best describes you.

In the following example, the circled 4 indicates the statement is not much like the person completing the assessment:

	Very Much Like Me	Usually Like Me	Somewhat Like Me	Not Like Me
When balancing work and leisure:				
1. I work most weekends and evenings	1	2	3	(4)

This is not a test and there are no right or wrong answers. Do not spend too much time thinking about your answers. Your initial response will likely be the most true for you. Be sure to respond to every statement.

(Turn to the next page and begin)

SECTION VI: LIFE SKILLS SCALE

Life Skills Scale

	Very Much Like Me	Usually Like Me	Somewhat Like Me	Not Like Me
When balancing work and leisure:				
1. I work most weekends and evenings	1	2	3	4
2. I have lots of leisure activities	4	3	2	1
3. I get bored when I am not working	1	2	3	4
4. I like to take days off	4	3	2	1
5. I feel guilty when I am not working	1	2	3	4
6. I am constantly thinking about work	1	2	3	4
7. I go into work even if I am sick	1	2	3	4
8. I am not worried about advancing in my career	4	3	2	1
9. I often do not take a lunch break while at work	1	2	3	4
10. I like to balance work and leisure	4	3	2	1
11. I am driven to perform better than everyone else at work	1	2	3	4
12. I often feel like I must drop everything else for my work	1	2	3	4

WORK / LEISURE BALANCE TOTAL = _____

	Very Much Like Me	Usually Like Me	Somewhat Like Me	Not Like Me
When managing my time:				
13. People say that I have "no sense of time"	1	2	3	4
14. I have a daily planner I carry with me	4	3	2	1
15. Being late does not bother me	1	2	3	4
16. I would be "lost" without a watch	4	3	2	1
17. I complete most tasks at the last minute	1	2	3	4
18. I am often too busy to enjoy life	1	2	3	4
19. I tend to put things off until later	1	2	3	4
20. I make time to enjoy healthy pleasures in my life	4	3	2	1
21. I take on more commitments than I have time for	1	2	3	4
22. I always seem to be in a hurry	1	2	3	4
23. I have plenty of time to spend with my friends	4	3	2	1
24. I am able to balance all of my life roles	4	3	2	1

TIME MANAGEMENT TOTAL = _____

(Continued on the next page)

SECTION VI: LIFE SKILLS SCALE

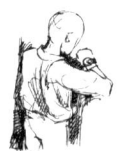

(Life Skills Scale Scale, continued)

When I am in a conflict with others:

25. I neglect my own wishes to satisfy the other person	1	2	3	4
26. I attempt to find a compromise	4	3	2	1
27. I give in so that I do not to hurt the other person's feelings	1	2	3	4
28. I accept the other person's position in exchange for the other person accepting mine	4	3	2	1
29. I postpone issues and think about them later	1	2	3	4
30. I attempt to get the other person to compromise	4	3	2	1
31. I do anything I can to get my way	1	2	3	4
32. I usually let others take responsibility for solving the problem	1	2	3	4
33. I do not like to give up my point of view	2	3	4	
34. I do what I can to avoid conflict	4	3	2	1
35. I always look for some way for all of us to win	4	3	2	1
36. I sacrifice my wants for those of others	1	2	3	4

CONFLICT RESOLUTION TOTAL = _____

When managing my money:

37. I buy whatever brings me pleasure	1	2	3	4
38. I have a hard time budgeting my money	1	2	3	4
39. It is difficult for me to save money	1	2	3	4
40. I buy things on impulse	1	2	3	4
41. I often overspend the money I earn	1	2	3	4
42. I am often in debt	1	2	3	4
43. I am great at saving money	4	3	2	1
44. I enjoy learning about and researching investments	4	3	2	1
45. I often buy non-essential items	1	2	3	4
46. I put a lot of time into managing my money	4	3	2	1
47. I spend a lot of emotional energy worrying about finances	1	2	3	4
48. I am focused on financial stability	4	3	2	1

MONEY MANAGEMENT TOTAL = _____

(Go to the Scoring Directions on the next page)

SECTION VI: LIFE SKILLS SCALE

Life Skills Scale
Scoring Directions

Four of the most important life skills that people need to develop are the ability to balance work and leisure, the ability to manage your time, the ability to resolve conflicts, and the ability to manage money. For each of the four sections on the previous pages, add the scores you circled. Put that total on the line marked "Total" at the end of each section.

Then, transfer your totals to the spaces below:

WORK / LEISURE BALANCE TOTAL = _____

TIME MANAGEMENT TOTAL = _____

CONFLICT RESOLUTION TOTAL = _____

MONEY MANAGEMENT TOTAL = _____

Profile Interpretation

Total Scales Score	Result	Indications
37 to 48	high	You have developed and you use many positive life skills in your daily life.
24 to 36	moderate	You have developed adequate life skills, but need to continue working to develop them even further.
12 to 23	low	It is very important for you to work on developing positive life skills for daily living.

For scales which you scored in the **Moderate** or **High** range, find the descriptions on the pages that follow. Then, read the description and complete the exercises that are included. No matter how you scored, low, moderate or high, you will benefit from these exercises.

Life Skills Scale Descriptions

Work / Leisure Balance

People who score low on this scale see their job as their greatest (and sometimes only) source of life satisfaction. They work long hours and devote much of their energy to their jobs, sometimes even preferring work to spending time with family and friends. As a consequence, they perform well in demanding jobs. Leisure may be important in their lives, but only after all their work is done. They are result-oriented and will often work extra hours to complete projects. They need work that is challenging, that allows them to set goals, and allows them to measure their achievement. They appreciate recognition and strive to get it. They often feel guilty when they are not working. Some might say they are addicted to the work they do.

Time Management

People who score low on this scale do not manage their time well. They probably put projects off till the last minute often because they are too busy or just because they are in the habit of procrastinating. They tend to always be in a hurry and are not able to balance relationships, work, school, and leisure. People with limited time management skills always feel they must be busy. They take on too many commitments and then are forced to do many different things at the same time. They feel driven and work hard to fulfill their obligations. Unfortunately, this leaves little time for leisure, friends, and family.

Conflict Resolution

People who score low on this scale are not willing to give up part of their goals in order to reach an agreement with another person in a conflict. They are willing to sacrifice part of their relationship with the other person in order to get their way. They do not believe in negotiating and trying to compromise in the situation so that both people get what they want. They are not willing to give a little to get a little. They are usually more concerned with having their way than they are with the feelings of the other person. No matter what the cost, winning it all is the most important to them.

Money Management

People who score low on this scale tend to get carried away by instant gratification in their life or simply do not have enough money on which they can survive. They often feel compelled to spend or charge money very easily and quickly, even if they can't afford the purchases. They will shop and spend compulsively and tend to buy things they do not need. They often have several credit cards, many of which might be charged to their limit. They may also not make enough money to be able purchase the essential life needs.

Work / Leisure Balance

For you to be happy and live a life that is mostly free of stress, you need to be able to balance work and leisure. Research has determined that a balanced combination of job satisfaction and leisure satisfaction is one of the primary predictors of physical and psychological health: Job satisfaction alone is not enough.

For many people, leisure is the *antidote* to a lack of job satisfaction. One of the ways that leisure can help people who are bored or lack meaning and satisfaction at work is through compensatory leisure activities. People who are unfulfilled at work can make up for it through hobbies and activities that satisfy the needs not being met on the job.

Ultimately, the relationship between your work and leisure, and the effects of the balance (or imbalance) between the two can take a variety of forms:

- **Separation:** Your work and leisure are two distinct facets of your life which do not influence each other. While possible, it is hard to imagine that the time put into work and the money earned from it have no impact on your hobbies or interests, or that leisure activities have no effect on your work life. One can be a social worker for a crisis center but make jewelry as a leisure activity. True separation may be quite difficult to manage but can be done.

List those times when your work and leisure activities are very *different* from each other.

_____
_____
_____
_____

- **Spillover:** There is little or no distinction between your work and leisure. You find so much satisfaction engaging in one activity that you choose to do it in both your work and leisure time. Imagine a veterinarian who loves working with animals so much that she volunteers at the local animal shelter on the weekends, or a video game designer who plays Xbox in his free time.

List those times when your work and leisure activities *spilled over* into each other.

_____
_____
_____
_____

(Continued on the next page)

(Work / Leisure Balance, continued)

- **Compensation:** What may be lacking in one arena of life can be compensated by satisfying activities in another. For example, someone who dislikes her desk job shuffles papers because it is too stationary and predictable, may enjoy mountain climbing on the weekends.

List those times when your work and leisure activities *compensated* for each other.

_____
_____
_____
_____

- **Conflict:** High levels of demand in one area of life can cause conflicts in the other. Such conflicts are frequent and are often part of the home / work balance process, although they can be avoided and managed. A person who is working too much may experience difficulties at home with family members — a common complaint among workers who feel the pressure to put their careers first.

List those times when your work and leisure activities *conflicted* with each other.

_____
_____
_____
_____

Recognizing the patterns that your work and leisure take, how they interact, and the effects that interaction has on your well being is key to identifying what you want out of your life work. Knowing the balance you need to strike can help you develop a plan that is right for you.

Ideas for Work / Leisure / Relationship Balance

In addition to simply choosing and engaging in your favorite leisure activities, there are other things you can do to have a more balanced life.

Consider the following as you seek to find your balance.

- **Time for relationships**

    It is important that you take time each day to connect with important people in your life. This may mean scheduling this time (actually writing it in a calendar or planner) until you begin to adopt it as a permanent part of your day.

- **Time alone**

    Take time for yourself. Use it to reflect and recharge. Try meditating for ten minutes a day and increasing the time as is comfortable for you. Meditation can help you focus on the moment and stop thinking about work that needs to be done in the future.

- **Breaks**

    You can easily build breaks into your work schedule. Even if you have been working quite well without taking breaks, you probably have not experienced your optimum level of creativity, motivation, and energy. Almost all employers allow for some breaks during the day.

- **Exercise**

    Exercise has been shown to be an excellent stress buster. People who exercise regularly tend to be happier, are more energetic, have a better outlook on life, and are able to cope much more effectively with stress.

- **Vacations**

    Use your vacation time for rest and relaxation. Of course everyone has a different idea about what constitutes rest and relaxation. Some people love sight-seeing vacations. Others prefer to rent a cabin on the lake only an hour out of town. The secret is to commit to using your vacation days (don't try to carry them over without a great reason for doing so) and finding a restful way to spend them.

SECTION VI: ACTIVITY HANDOUTS

Time Management

There are many different ways in which you can manage your time more effectively.

Some of these techniques include:

Letting Go of the Guilts

What do you feel obligated to do ... or think that you 'should' do?

_____
_____
_____
_____

Now turn those obligations or 'shoulds' into CHOICES:

_____
_____
_____
_____

Delegate Responsibilities at Work and at Home

What sorts of things are you doing that don't require your personal attention?

_____
_____
_____
_____

To whom could you delegate?

_____
_____
_____
_____

(Continued on the next page)

(Time Management, continued)

Reassess the Activities You Engage In

Describe your activities in a typical day (include work, school, family, parenting, etc.):

_____
_____

What changes can you make to have more free time for yourself?

_____
_____

Make Time for Yourself

How can you manage your time to re-energize yourself? When during the day could you find time to relax or meditate?

_____
_____

Don't Be Afraid to Say "No"

In what types of situations do you find yourself saying "yes" when you want to say "no?"

_____
_____

Why do you find yourself saying "yes" in these situations? To whom do you say it?

_____
_____

What types of commitments and obligations do you take on that are not necessary?

_____
_____

Conflict Resolution

Conflict is an evitable part of everyone's life. Conflict resolution is a social skill that is important for your personal growth and development. People who are successful in life are able to effectively resolve conflict. For effective conflict resolution, it is important to identify the situations which create conflict in your life. The following chart will help you to learn more about where and when most of your conflicts occur.

Where and When My Conflicts Occur

List with whom most of your conflicts occur (a neighbor, significant other, co-workers, friends, parents, etc.) and when most of your conflicts occur (after a hard day at work, when your children act out, when your significant other does not listen to what you are saying, when your parents make unreasonable demands on you, etc.).

With whom conflicts occur	When the conflicts occur

SECTION VI: ACTIVITY HANDOUTS

Conflict Resolution Patterns

List some conflicts that you have had in your life.

What strategies did you use and what might have been a better solution to the conflict?

Conflicts I remember	How the conflict was resolved	A better solution might have been

What patterns do you see emerging?

_____

_____

_____

Money Matters

Money management is very difficult for most people. We tend to have a lot of different emotions about money. Some people love it, worship it, fear it, hate it, don't understand it, simply accept it for what it is or just never have enough. However, managing the money we have is often a problem for many people. Managing your money and developing a financial plan can be very difficult if you do not understand your own reactions to money.

If you spend more money than you have, what do you think causes you to do this?

_____

_____

If you overspend, what do you think are the deep-seated roots to your overspending?

_____

_____

How does your money history affect the way you overspend?

_____

_____

What emotional or psychological voids does spending money fill?

_____

_____

What effect has your childhood and your parents spending habits had on you?

_____

_____

How does spending money make you feel?

_____

_____

How does not having enough money make you feel?

_____

_____

What could you do if you do not have enough money to meet your obligations?

_____

_____

SECTION V: ACTIVITY HANDOUTS

Family Monthly Budget Worksheet

This worksheet is designed to help you determine the approximate amount of money you spend each month and where you might be able to save more money:

MONTHLY EXPENSES	CURRENT AMOUNT PAID
Rent or Mortgage	$_____
Car Payment	$_____
TV/Cable	$_____
Loan Repayment	$_____
Medical/Dental Expenses	$_____
Insurance (Life, Auto, Home, Medical)	$_____
Credit Card Payments	$_____
Clothing	$_____
Education	$_____
Automobile Expenses	$_____
Parking/Gas	$_____
Groceries	$_____
Entertainment	$_____
Restaurants / Coffee Shops	$_____
Allowances	$_____
Telephone Bill	$_____
Gas and Electricity	$_____
Water and Sewage	$_____
Sanitation	$_____
Household Repairs	$_____
Taxes (State, Local, Federal)	$_____
Child Care	$_____
Newspaper, Books or Magazines	$_____
Eating Out	$_____
Hobbies	$_____
Unpaid old bills	$_____
Other	$_____
TOTAL MONTHLY EXPENSES =	**$**_____
TOTAL MONTHLY SAVINGS =	**$**_____

What expenses are not necessary and could be reduced or eliminated to help you save more money each month?

_____

_____

_____

SECTION VI: JOURNALING ACTIVITIES

I learned . . .

The most important things I learned about how I **balance work and leisure** . . .

(Continued on the next page)

SECTION V: JOURNALING ACTIVITIES

I learned . . .

The most important things I learned about how I **manage my time** . . .

(Continued on the next page)

SECTION VI: JOURNALING ACTIVITIES

I learned . . .

The most important things I learned about how I **manage conflicts** . . .

(Continued on the next page)

SECTION V: JOURNALING ACTIVITIES

I learned . . .

The most important things I learned about how I **manage my money** . . .

Positive Life Skills

- Empower you to manage daily living effectively

- Empower you to create order and stability in your life

- Empower you to take responsibility for your own wellness

- Empower you to grow personally and professionally

- Empower you to balance daily priorities

- Empower you to overcome and accept your past and go forward with confidence

- Empower you create the future you deserve

Whole Person Associates is the leading publisher of training resources for professionals who empower people to create and maintain healthy lifestyles. Our creative resources will help you work effectively with your clients in the areas of stress management, wellness promotion, mental health and life skills.

Please visit us at our web site: **www.wholeperson.com**. You can check out our entire line of products, place an order, request our print catalog, and sign up for our monthly special notifications.

Whole Person Associates

800-247-6789